CHAIR PILA

SENIORS

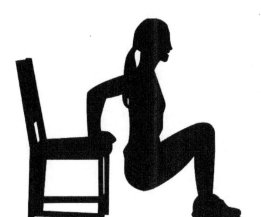

A Step-by-Step Guide to Rejuvenate your

Body and Mind with Easy Workouts

CARMEN GRACEFIELD

Copyright © 2023 by Carmen Gracefield

This book is intended for informational purposes only and should not be considered a substitute for professional medical advice, diagnosis, or treatment. Always consult with a qualified healthcare provider before beginning any exercise program or making significant changes to your lifestyle. The author disclaims any liability arising directly or indirectly from the use of the exercises, techniques, or information contained in this book.

Contents

INTRODUCTION

In the quiet corners of life, where memories and wisdom intertwine, there exists a realm of cherished moments that have shaped the journey of our golden years. As we age, our bodies may wear the badges of time, but our spirits remain ever-vibrant, eager to embrace new experiences and challenges. It is within this spirit that we embark on a transformative voyage through the pages of "Chair Pilates for Seniors."

Imagine a quaint little town nestled between rolling hills and meandering streams. In this town lived a remarkable woman named Eleanor. Her silvery hair held stories of decades gone by, and her eyes twinkled with the light of a life well-lived. But beneath the surface, Eleanor was grappling with the silent challenges that often accompany the passage of years – the stiffening of joints, the loss of balance, and the yearning for vitality.

One day, as the sun painted the sky with hues of amber and gold, Eleanor's curiosity led her to a local community center. There, she encountered a group of seniors engaged in a seemingly magical practice. Seated comfortably in chairs, they moved with grace and purpose, their bodies swaying in gentle harmony. This was Chair Pilates – a haven of rejuvenation that was about to change Eleanor's life.

With each session, Eleanor's muscles rediscovered their suppleness, her posture improved, and her sense of balance became steadfast. But it was not just her physical being that underwent a transformation. As her body flowed through the fluid motions of Chair Pilates, Eleanor found solace in her mind. Her worries seemed to melt away, replaced by a serene sense of presence.

As you hold this book in your hands, dear reader, you are embarking on a similar journey. Within these pages, you will find an array of easy-to-follow Chair Pilates exercises tailored to embrace the needs and aspirations of older men and women. Whether you're a seasoned Pilates enthusiast or someone taking their first steps into the realm of mindful movement, this book is your guide to rediscovering the joy of physical activity while honoring the unique needs of your body.

Through clear instructions, detailed illustrations, and a wealth of insights, "Chair Pilates for Seniors" empowers you to embark on a path of holistic well-being. As you embrace the gentle stretches, mindful breaths, and graceful movements, you will not only enhance your physical vitality but also nurture your emotional resilience.

So, let us embark on this transformative journey together, where the chair becomes not just a piece of furniture but a vessel of strength, grace, and renewal. Just as Eleanor found her haven amidst the flowing movements of Chair Pilates, you too will discover a sanctuary of wellness that celebrates the beauty and wisdom of your golden years.

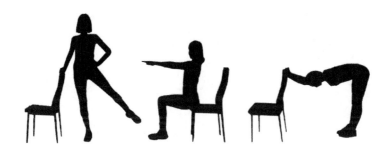

CHAIR PILATES EXERCISES TAILORED FOR SENIORS

Here are some easy Chair Pilates exercises tailored for seniors. Remember to consult with a healthcare professional before starting any new exercise routine, especially if you have any existing health conditions.

1. Seated March:

- Sit tall in the chair with your feet flat on the floor.
- Lift one knee towards your chest and then lower it.
- Alternate legs, creating a marching motion.
- Repeat for 20-30 marches on each leg.

2. Seated Twist:

- Sit tall with your feet flat on the floor and hands resting on your thighs.

- Inhale and as you exhale, twist your upper body to the right, using your left hand to gently push against your right thigh for resistance.
- Hold for a few breaths, then repeat on the other side.
- Perform 5-7 twists on each side.

3. Leg Extensions:

- Sit tall with your feet flat on the floor.
- Extend one leg forward, keeping it straight.
- Flex your foot and hold for a few seconds, then point your toes and hold.
- Lower your foot back to the floor.
- Alternate legs and repeat for 10-15 extensions on each leg.

4. Seated Cat-Cow Stretch:

- Sit tall with your hands resting on your thighs.

- Inhale as you arch your back, lifting your chest and looking up (Cow pose).

- Exhale as you round your back, tucking your chin to your chest (Cat pose).

- Repeat the sequence, flowing between Cow and Cat poses for 5-7 rounds.

5. Seated Shoulder Rolls:

- Sit tall and relax your arms by your sides.

- Inhale as you lift your shoulders towards your ears.

- Exhale as you roll your shoulders back and down.

- Repeat for 10-15 rounds, then switch directions and roll your shoulders forward and up.

6. Ankle Circles:

- Sit tall with your feet flat on the floor.
- Lift one foot off the ground and gently rotate your ankle in circles.
- Perform 5-7 circles in each direction, then switch to the other ankle.

7. Seated Side Stretch:

- Sit tall with your feet flat on the floor and your arms by your sides.
- Inhale and raise your left arm overhead.
- Exhale and gently lean to the right, feeling a stretch along your left side.
- Inhale to return to the center and switch sides.
- Perform 3-5 stretches on each side.

Remember to breathe deeply and move slowly and mindfully during these exercises. If you experience any discomfort or pain, stop immediately. Chair

Pilates is designed to promote flexibility, strength, and relaxation, so enjoy the benefits of these gentle movements at your own pace.

8. Seated Chest Opener:

- Sit tall with your feet flat on the floor and your hands resting on your lap.
- Inhale and interlace your fingers behind your back, pressing your palms together.
- Exhale and gently lift your arms away from your body, opening your chest.
- Hold for a few breaths, then release.
- Repeat 3-5 times.

9. Seated Leg Lifts:

- Sit tall with your feet flat on the floor and hands on the armrests.
- Inhale and lift one leg off the floor, extending it forward.

- Exhale and lower the leg back down.
- Alternate legs and repeat for 10-15 leg lifts on each side.

10. Seated Spinal Twist with Arm Reach:

- Sit tall with your feet flat on the floor and your arms by your sides.
- Inhale and lift your right arm overhead.
- Exhale and twist your upper body to the left, reaching your right hand towards the left side of the chair.
- Inhale to return to the center and switch sides.
- Perform 3-5 twists on each side.

11. Seated Hip Circles:

- Sit tall with your feet flat on the floor.
- Place your hands on your hips and gently circle your hips in a clockwise direction.

- After a few circles, switch to counterclockwise.
- Perform 5-7 circles in each direction.

12. Seated Shoulder Stretch:

- Sit tall and extend your right arm straight out in front of you at shoulder height.
- Use your left hand to gently press the back of your right hand, stretching your shoulder.
- Hold for a few breaths, then switch sides.
- Repeat 3-5 times on each side.

13. Seated Toe Taps:

- Sit tall with your feet flat on the floor.
- Lift your toes off the ground while keeping your heels on the floor.
- Tap your toes back down, then lift your heels while keeping your toes on the ground.
- Repeat the sequence for 20-30 taps.

- Sit tall and gently tilt your head to the right, bringing your right ear towards your right shoulder.
- Hold for a few breaths, then return to the center and tilt your head to the left.
- Repeat on each side 3-5 times.

These Chair Pilates exercises offer a well-rounded approach to improving flexibility, mobility, and overall well-being. Remember to listen to your body, and only do what feels comfortable. Regular practice of these gentle movements can help seniors maintain their physical and mental vitality, while also fostering a sense of connection between the body and mind.

15. Seated Side Leg Lifts:

- Sit tall with your feet flat on the floor and your hands on the armrests.
- Inhale and lift one leg out to the side, keeping it straight.
- Exhale and lower the leg back down.
- Alternate legs and repeat for 10-15 leg lifts on each side.

16. Seated Ankle Flexes:

- Sit tall with your feet flat on the floor.
- Lift one foot off the ground and flex your ankle, pointing your toes toward the ceiling.
- Release and point your toes away from you.
- Alternate ankle flexes for 10-15 reps on each foot.

17. Seated Arm Circles:

- Sit tall with your feet flat on the floor and arms extended out to the sides at shoulder height.
- Inhale as you circle your arms forward, bringing your palms to touch in front of you.
- Exhale as you circle your arms out to the sides and then back behind you.
- Repeat for 10-15 arm circles.

18. Seated Pelvic Tilts:

- Sit tall with your feet flat on the floor.
- Inhale and tilt your pelvis forward, arching your lower back slightly.
- Exhale and tilt your pelvis backward, rounding your lower back.
- Repeat the pelvic tilts, moving with your breath, for 10-15 rounds.

19. Seated Wrist Stretches:

- Sit tall with your arms extended forward at shoulder height.
- Flex your wrists so that your fingers point towards the ceiling.
- Hold for a few breaths, then release and point your fingers toward the floor.
- Repeat 3-5 times for each wrist.

20. Seated Deep Breathing:

- Sit tall with your hands resting on your lap.
- Inhale deeply through your nose, expanding your belly.
- Exhale slowly through your mouth, letting go of any tension.
- Focus on the rhythm of your breath and repeat for 5-10 deep breaths.

These Chair Pilates exercises continue to provide a gentle and effective way for seniors to engage in mindful movement and maintain their overall well-being. Regular practice can help improve circulation, flexibility, and muscle strength, while also promoting relaxation and reducing stress. Remember to perform these exercises in a comfortable and safe manner, and feel free to modify them as needed to suit your individual needs and abilities.

IMMUNE-BOOSTING RECIPES SUITABLE FOR SENIORS

Here are a few immune-boosting and nutritious recipes that are suitable for seniors:

1. Immune-Boosting Breakfast Smoothie:

Ingredients:

- 1 cup fresh spinach
- 1/2 cup frozen berries (blueberries, strawberries, or mixed berries)
- 1 small banana
- 1/2 cup Greek yogurt (or non-dairy alternative)
- 1 tablespoon chia seeds
- 1/2 cup water or unsweetened almond milk

Instructions: Blend all ingredients until smooth and creamy. Pour into a glass and enjoy this nutrient-packed start to your day.

2. Quinoa and Vegetable Salad:

Ingredients:

- 1 cup cooked quinoa
- 1 cup mixed vegetables (e.g., bell peppers, cucumbers, cherry tomatoes, carrots), chopped
- 1/4 cup chopped fresh herbs (such as parsley, basil, or mint)
- 2 tablespoons olive oil
- 1 tablespoon lemon juice
- Salt and pepper to taste

Instructions: In a bowl, combine the cooked quinoa, mixed vegetables, and fresh herbs. Drizzle with olive oil and lemon juice, and season with salt and pepper. Toss well to combine and serve as a refreshing and nutritious salad.

3. Baked Salmon with Garlic and Herbs:

Ingredients:

- 2 salmon fillets
- 2 cloves garlic, minced
- 1 tablespoon fresh lemon juice
- 1 tablespoon chopped fresh dill or thyme
- Salt and pepper to taste

Instructions: Preheat the oven to 375°F (190°C). Place salmon fillets on a baking sheet lined with parchment paper. In a small bowl, mix minced garlic, lemon juice, chopped herbs, salt, and pepper. Spread the garlic and herb mixture evenly over the salmon fillets. Bake in the preheated oven for about 15-20 minutes or until salmon is cooked through and flakes easily with a fork.

Ingredients:

- 1 cup milk (dairy or non-dairy)
- 1/2 teaspoon ground turmeric
- 1/4 teaspoon ground cinnamon
- 1/4 teaspoon ground ginger
- 1 teaspoon honey (optional)

Instructions: In a small saucepan, heat the milk over low heat. Add turmeric, cinnamon, and ginger. Whisk to combine. Heat the mixture until it's warmed through, but not boiling. Remove from heat, add honey if desired, and stir well. Pour into a mug and enjoy this comforting immune-boosting drink.

These recipes are designed to be flavorful, easy to prepare, and packed with nutrients to support seniors' overall health and well-being.

CONCLUSION: EMBRACE YOUR GOLDEN JOURNEY

As you reach the end of this transformative journey through "Chair Pilates for Seniors" take a moment to reflect on the path you've embarked upon. You've delved into the world of mindful movement, discovering the power that lies within gentle stretches, graceful poses, and conscious breaths.

Throughout these pages, we've explored the harmony between the body and mind, recognizing that age is but a number and the spirit knows no bounds. The chair has become your companion, a steadfast ally on your quest for strength, flexibility, and well-being. You've embraced each exercise with curiosity, and in doing so, you've rekindled the flame of vitality that resides within.

Remember, this journey doesn't end here. It is a continuum, a dance that you'll carry with you as you navigate the chapters yet to come. Chair Pilates has become more than a series of movements; it's a philosophy of self-care, a testament to the enduring relationship between movement and wellness.

As you move forward, keep your heart open to the possibilities that lie ahead. Let each breath remind you of the innate resilience of your body, and let each stretch serve as a celebration of the life you've lived and the life still unfolding before you. Share your newfound wisdom with those around you, for your journey is an inspiration to others seeking to embrace the fullness of their golden years.

In the company of your chair, you've discovered a sanctuary of rejuvenation, a place where the body and mind harmonize, and where time becomes a canvas for your continued growth. Cherish this gift you've given yourself, and carry it forward with gratitude and grace.

Thank you for embarking on this journey with us. May your days be filled with the joy of movement, the embrace of well-being, and the unwavering spirit of a life well-lived.

With warmest regards,

Carmen Gracefield

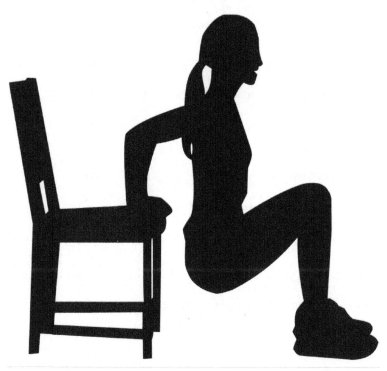

Printed in Great Britain
by Amazon